BRAIN-BALANCE
WORKOUT

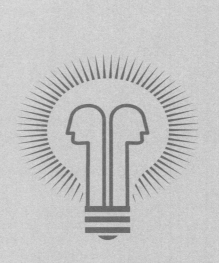

BRAIN-BALANCE
WORKOUT

50 puzzles to change the
way you think

CHARLES PHILLIPS

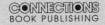

CONNECTIONS
BOOK PUBLISHING

For Thomas David Phillips

A CONNECTIONS EDITION
This edition published in Great Britain in 2013 by
Connections Book Publishing Limited
St Chad's House, 148 King's Cross Road, London WC1X 9DH
www.connections-publishing.com

British Library Cataloguing-in-Publication data available on request.

ISBN 978-1-85906-378-1

1   3   5   7   9   10   8   6   4   2

Phototypeset in Cafeteria and Vectora LH using InDesign on Apple Macintosh
Printed in Singapore

CONTENTS

Introduction

Are you sometimes surprised by the decisions you take? You know what you *think* you should do, what the logical choice is, but somehow you find yourself driven to go for another option— because it feels right or perhaps because your instincts or intuitions tell you to do it.

Or, do you sometimes find you're completely stuck on a problem, then an answer suddenly comes to you, as if from nowhere?

This contrast between logic and instinct, reason and intuition, conscious and unconscious decision-making derives from your thinking organ's division into left and right brain.

A brain of two halves The upper brain is divided into two regions: the left and right hemispheres. Neuroscientists report that in the right hemisphere your brain maintains awareness of the background and how things connect, while in the left, information-processing focuses on the foreground and detail.

Traditionally, some researchers have broadened the distinction, identifying the left brain as the home of logical analysis, of mathematics and language use, and the right brain as the home of creative insight, artistic and musical abilities. In this outlook, the left side is associated with detail and intellectual thought, and the right with the "big picture," with instinct and emotions.

Moments of insight In his book *Imagine: How Creativity Works*, Jonah Lehrer discusses how moments of insight are preceded by impasse—a sense that your thinking about a problem has no productive outlet, that you cannot reach an answer. He describes tests carried out by psychologists Mark Beeman and John Kounios which suggested that, while your conscious attempts to solve a problem are principally conducted in your left brain, you rely on your right brain for the wider connections, the metaphorical, more associative thinking that feeds into moments of insight.

The tests focused on volunteers attempting to solve a word problem while being monitored both by electroencephalography (EEG), which tracks mental activity as embodied by brainwaves, and by an fMRI machine (a brain scanner that identifies brain activity through bloodflow). Beeman and Kounios found that when you try to solve a word problem your brain initially works through possible solutions; at this point there is increased activity in areas of the left brain associated with speech and language. Sometimes this search succeeds, and you come up with the answer. If the search fails, however, you have the familiar sense of an impasse—which may be followed by a swift insight.

Just before you become consciously aware of the insight, there is sudden high activity in an area of the right brain called the anterior superior temporal gyrus (aSTG), situated just above the right ear and linked by other studies to understanding literary themes and metaphors. This is followed by a burst of gamma brainwaves, high-frequency waves associated by neuroscientists with binding cells in a new network of connections. Without you being conscious of the process, your brain makes new links that furnish you with the insight—the answer.

Once the insight arrives, you know it's right. At this point your prefrontal cortex shows enhanced activity. This is the front upper part of the brain, associated with abstract reasoning, and with monitoring and managing the activities of other brain parts.

Thinking styles We each have a unique thinking style. This is a product of both nature and nurture: on the one hand—our genetic makeup; on the other—how we were cared for in infancy, how we fared in school and college, how we set about managing our mental life and further educating ourselves in later years.

To improve your decision-making, you need to have a good sense of your natural thinking style. The key thing: Try to balance your thinking—not to eliminate emotions and instincts, but to be aware of how they influence your decisions. The aim is not to elevate the left brain above the right brain, or the right brain above the left brain, but to balance the two. And that's where this book comes in. The left-brain/right-brain distinction is an engaging and fun way to characterize different outlooks on the world, as well as identifying your strengths, and improving your thinking.

How the book works First, try Thinking Challenge 1 (pages 11–14), designed to test your thinking style in a real-life scenario, then check pages 92–3 to see how you fared. Next, answer the Left-Brain/Right-Brain Questionnaire (page 15) to learn how your thinking is currently balanced. Work out your total Starting Score (see page 93), then begin with Left or Right Puzzle 1.

Creativity versus language

Research in 2010 suggested that brain regions for language and creativity are in competition with one another—and this may explain the remarkable finding that people who suffer left-brain damage often become more creative. The research, led by Simone Shamay-Tsoory at the University of Haifa, Israel, studied people with damage to one of three brain regions. Those who had damage in a region of the left hemisphere associated with language use scored more highly for creativity than those with no damage. The people who scored lowest for creativity had damage in part of the right hemisphere believed to be crucial for decision-making and planning. The report suggested that creativity in the right hemisphere may be suppressed by language areas of the left brain, but that when these left-brain areas are damaged, creativity increases.

Proceed now through the fifty puzzles, which are intended to develop your skills in typically left-brain processes, such as logical thought, and typically right-brain processes, for instance spatial perception. Difficulty levels range from 1 to 5, so you can be sure your brain will be stretched to the limit. After each puzzle, to find out where to go next, score yourself between 0 and 5, depending on whether you got the answer right and how easy you found it (from 0 for very hard and incorrect, to 5 for very easy and correct).

• **Scores of 0, 1, or 2** lead to a puzzle of the same kind.
• **Scores of 3, 4, or 5** lead to a puzzle of the other kind.

For example, if you start with Left Puzzle 1 and score 3, 4, or 5, indicating a degree of success, proceed to Right Puzzle 1. But if you score 0, 1, or 2, indicating that you struggled with it to some extent, proceed to Left Puzzle 2. You always proceed to the next question in the numerical L or R sequence. So, you might proceed like this: L1–L2–L3–R1–L4–R2–R3–R4–L5. Or like this: R1–R2–R3–R4–R5–L1–R6–L2–L3. (You don't need to total up your scores as you work through the book—they're only there to tell you where to go next—but do mark them so you can judge your performance at the end. See page 94 for guidance.)

The aim is to attempt all fifty puzzles, so if you do all the Left puzzles using the process described above, you then proceed through the remaining Right puzzles in numerical order; likewise, if you complete all the Right puzzles, proceed through the remaining Left puzzles in numerical order. Finally, take the climactic **Thinking Challenge 2** to gauge your progress overall.

Once you've worked your way through the book, you'll be well on your way to fine-tuning your brain and learning how to think *better*. You have a whole brain—now use it!

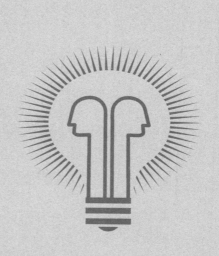

THINKING CHALLENGE 1

The following pages give you the chance to assess your thinking style, which—as we've seen—depends on the relative strengths of your right-brain and left-brain conceptualizing. Perhaps you're strong at visual thinking and can swiftly see a solution to a problem, or maybe you prefer to progress slowly and steadily through data when working toward an answer. Do you always think things through logically before you make a choice? Or do you sometimes make decisions based on your intuition rather than on immediately available facts?

Work through the thinking challenge "In Bloom" on pages 12–14, then respond to the questionnaire on page 15. This challenge is designed to put left-brain/right-brain differences and choices in an entertaining, real-life-scenario context, and is complemented by questions that focus on your likely response to a variety of everyday situations. This works best if you answer honestly—describe how you actually think, rather than how you wish you could think.

Then turn to pages 92–3 for guidance on scoring and assessing your response, before starting on the puzzles. Good luck!

In Bloom

Your arms are full of flowers. Today you're starting a new job. You've been laid off from a demanding position at Rainbow Productions, a large broadcasting company; in the end, after surviving many redundancy cycles, your departure came as something of a relief. But of course times are tough, and new jobs are few and far between—so you're delighted when family friend Joy offers you the chance to be a delivery driver and all-round assistant at her shop, Joy Blooms, a high-end florist. You're ready for a new challenge … and determined that you'll succeed at this.

Your first task is to make a delivery of several potted trees and plants to a valued client, Dame Helen Somerville, who lives in the Ocean View Hotel at 210 Vine Parade. This order is running late, and must arrive in time for a video call she is making to a theater director in London in the UK—so you have to be efficient and prompt.

Notes

Unfortunately, the GPS in your delivery van is malfunctioning. The following instructions are read to you over your cellphone: From the shop on Ridgeway Avenue, go north to the offices of Screen World, right on Oyster Way, at St. Nicholas Cathedral take a left along Yale Crescent, go right at the Theodore Roosevelt statue, through the underpass at Green Circle, right beside the Méliès Movie Theater along Berwick Way, left at the supermarket onto Inglewood, then right at the Viking Hotel onto Vine Parade.

How would you go about memorizing these instructions? You have only 10 minutes to get the bouquet to Dame Helen.

The second job is to build a new display shelf at the front of the shop. Joy is always cost-conscious and has purchased the unit, which is made by a well-known manufacturer, at a knockdown price. You have the product code but no assembly instructions. She asks you to get it finished within the hour because a buyer from a major department store is dropping in before noon and she needs the shop to look its best.

Notes

The third job of the day requires you to deliver lilies to reclusive multimillionaire Hermann Caine, which involves another trip to Vine, the upscale section of town. Gaining access to Caine's penthouse apartment isn't straightforward, however: You have to key three entry codes into three successive security doors. Joy explains that this is a requirement of the contract: Caine has fired all his security and reception staff and insists on electronic security only.

The codes are 14789 at the outer door, 159753 at the lobby door, and 7415369 at the apartment door. To help you memorize them, she suggests you try closing your eyes and visualizing a hand entering the numbers on a keypad.

Finally, you're asked to step in and make up a series of bouquets for your old broadcasting company, who need them for the set of a new sitcom—based in a florist's store!

(Turn to pages 92–3 for guidance on scoring and to find out how to assess your responses on this and the questions opposite.)

Notes

Left-Brain/Right-Brain Questionnaire

Tick the answers that ring true, then turn to page 93 to find out your Starting Score.

AGREE

1. At work or college I'm often the one people turn to to find fresh ways to do things.

2. I prefer to think strategically rather than get involved in step-by-step processes.

3. If I have to cook an unfamiliar meal, I like to follow the instructions carefully and to the letter.

4. I quickly have a good sense of the best way to fit bags in the trunk of a car.

5. People turn to me if they want to settle disputes about sports stats or movie dates.

6. After I meet new people, I'm better at remembering names than faces.

7. I'd say I prefer geometry to algebra.

8. I wish people would speak plainly—I get confused by flowery language and sarcasm.

9. If I'm sorting out change, I prefer to look at the coins rather than write down figures.

10. I love doing sudoku and number puzzles, but I have to try harder to enjoy mazes.

THE PUZZLES

These fifty puzzles are designed to test typical areas of left-brain or right-brain processing. On the basis of how well you do, and how easy you find them, you can plot your own way through the book. If you're proving yourself strong in right-brain thinking, you'll be directed to questions that develop typically left-brain skills—and vice versa—with the aim of developing a balanced thinking style. Handy Thinking Tips are included throughout, to help you improve your overall mental performance. Engage with the puzzles as positively as you can. Be alert to changes in your confidence and performance—and enjoy!

(Turn to page 9 if you need a reminder of how to score yourself as you progress through the book.)

Casino Dice

Virgil is a technician on a casino heist movie. Waiting to shoot a dice gambling sequence, he draws up this grid puzzle. Can you solve it? The challenge is to fill in the grid so that dice numbering 1–6 appear in all the rows and all the columns.

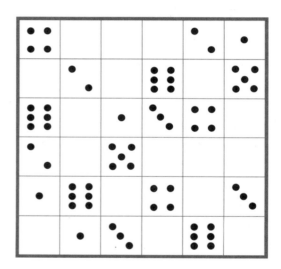

THINKING TIP
If you feel daunted by the effort involved in learning a new skill or breaking a bad habit, remember you have enormous capacity to change. Your brain makes 1 million new connections among its neurons every second.

Taking It Easy

City cycle couriers "Tricky" and "Easy" communicate by leaving one another route puzzles at the dispatch office. Here's one with sixteen stars and fourteen circles that Tricky made to mark Easy's thirtieth birthday. Can you complete it? The task is to find your way from A to B without passing through any circles, then make your way back from B to A without passing through any stars.

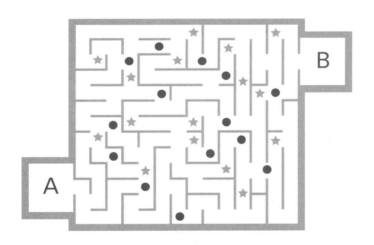

THINKING TIP
Try to approach puzzles—and indeed all challenges—in a positive frame of mind. If you're convinced you're not up to the task, you're more likely to fail.

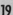

Firenze

In Alexandra's historical novel *Firenze*, Paolo is an apprentice in the workshop of a master painter and finds this small number puzzle among his master's papers. The task is to complete the grid so that the numbers 1–25 are all present, and all rows and columns add up to the totals indicated on the outside of the grid. In the plot of *Firenze*, Paolo has to solve the puzzle to discover the missing number from the center—the key to finding his lost sister Lucia.

2	16	24	3		62
12		11		19	61
	5		20	6	62
7		14	13		74
	9	23			66
50	67	82	65	61	

THINKING TIP
Practice makes you numerate. To boost your confidence with numbers, look out for everyday opportunities to do mental arithmetic.

Colors Fade

Gerard produced this design sketch during preproduction on the movie *Colors Fade*, a film about a mathematician who loses the ability to see in color. The design is for a dream sequence in which the lead character is agonizing over her reduced options. Can you work out what the ninth section should be—A, B, C, or D? All rows and columns must contain the same elements.

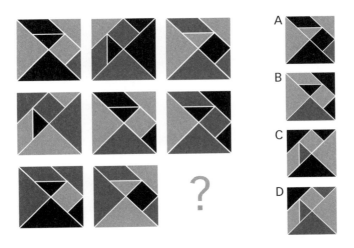

THINKING TIP
Brain scientists report that there are benefits in letting your mind wander—especially if you're in need of an insight to solve a seemingly intractable problem.

YOUR
SCORE

Sir Hector's Code

Longtime pals Sir Hector and Sir Jeremy often stroll on the sea-front at Bexhill-on-Sea, southern England, discussing their days in the diplomatic service. Sir Hector found this code puzzle in his attic and the old boys are trying to solve it. Can you help them? The letters are valued 1–26 according to their place in the alphabet (A = 1, B = 2, and so on): Your task is to crack the mystery code and reveal the missing letter.

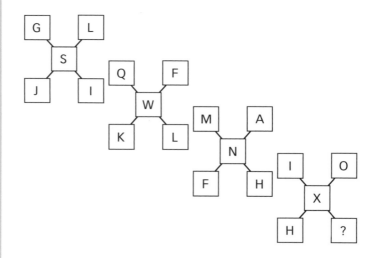

YOUR
SCORE

THINKING TIP
Try new things. Alter your routine, and make the most of your natural curiosity—Albert Einstein is reported to have said, "I have no particular talent, I am merely inquisitive."

Ransom

Physics student Suraj is playing a new video game, "Ransom": He has been kidnapped and stuck with several other prisoners in a warehouse. To escape he has to draw walls to partition the warehouse floor into areas, so that each area contains two prisoners (represented by squares). Area sizes must match those shown below the grid and each + must be linked to at least two walls.

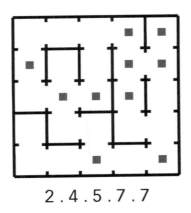

2 . 4 . 5 . 7 . 7

THINKING TIP
You can sometimes generate new ideas and gain fresh perspectives if you sketch a problem in visual form.

YOUR
SCORE

23

The Joy of Math

Grace, a retired mathematics teacher, introduced paper number-sum grids on all the tables when she began managing The Golden Oldies comedy club. Here's one of her puzzles. Can you solve it? The task is to use the numbers below to complete these six sums (three reading across and three downward). Each number is used once, and one—the 9—is already in place.

1 2 3 4 5 6 7 8 9

	+		−		=	4
−	■	x	■	+		
	+	9	−		=	6
x	■	+	■	−		
	+		x		=	22
=		=		=		
42		32		9		

THINKING TIP
Try meditation for clearer thinking. Research suggests the practice produces measurable improvements in both concentration and working memory. (See Further Reading & Resources on page 95 for more details.)

Path of Attraction

Fine art students Bernard and Heather met and fell in love working at the city garden center. Now each year Heather draws Bernard a floral card for Valentine's Day, and this year's card contains a puzzle, as shown: A butterfly is attracted to twenty flowers in a meadow in turn; you can see the end of her trip, but can you work out which flower was the first one she visited?

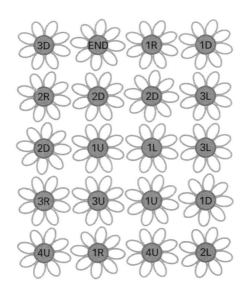

3D	END	1R	1D
2R	2D	2D	3L
2D	1U	1L	3L
3R	3U	1U	1D
4U	1R	4U	2L

THINKING TIP
A good time to generate insights is during the first few moments of the day, when you're just waking up … Why not set the alarm early to give yourself time to think before you have to get up and get on?

Whodunit?

Screenwriter Gilbert has a collection of these loopline puzzles that he completes for relaxation when he is working on Whodunit? plots. The task is to draw a single loop using horizontal and vertical lines only (the lines in some cells may turn 90 degrees; for example, head up then take a right turn). The loop must not pass through any cell more than once; any cell that the loop does not visit must be shaded in; no shaded cells can touch in either a horizontal or vertical direction (so the cells around shaded squares must all be part of the loop). Numbers with arrows (clue squares) indicate how many shaded cells appear in a given direction in a specific row or column; clue squares should be left untouched and do not form part of the loop, nor are they to be shaded in. Lastly, not all shaded cells are necessarily identified with arrows.

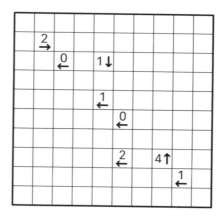

THINKING TIP
Play around with numbers and relations between numbers. You never know when you may need to perform a quick mental calculation, and being confident to do so is often the key to seeming smart and well informed.

A Symbol Problem

Jensen, a mathematician, took a stained-glass workshop in an attempt to balance his left/right thinking patterns. He came up with this design for a symbol window, in which a single part is missing from the grid. "Can you see how the part fits within the whole?" he asks his girlfriend Sarah. "Which of these four options below completes the grid if you place it in the empty space?"

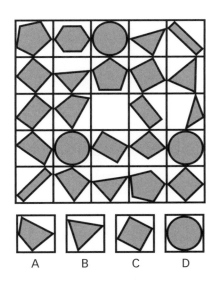

A   B   C   D

THINKING TIP
Try working on problems with friends. As long as the group works together harmoniously, you're all likely to benefit from fresh perspectives and approaches you didn't previously see.

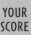

YOUR SCORE

Davy's Dice

Back on the set of the casino heist movie (see Left Puzzle 1), character actor Wilson Davy has made a contribution to the dice and playing-card puzzles that are being passed around by the crew. In Wilson's version, each shade (black, dark gray, light gray, or white) represents a direction (up, down, left, or right) and the number of dots on each die tell you how far to go. Starting in the middle die of the maze, follow the directions correctly and you will stop at every die in turn once only. If you do this, which die is the last you visit on your trip?

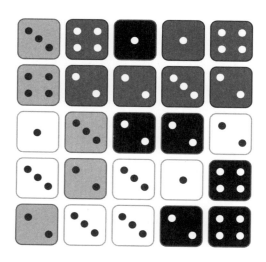

THINKING TIP
Try to be open to the unexpected—surprises can be mentally stimulating. In the twenty-first century our choices can be limited or routines directed by software that suggests what to buy or where to go.

Jigsaw Aria

In a new opera about British mathematicians, Roddy and Benedict—two members of the chorus—have to complete the giant puzzle shown below during the tenor's jokey "Jigsaw Aria." They had almost completed the puzzle, but the mischievous stage manager Jonathan has muddled up all the pieces. Can you help Roddy and Ben pick the four correct pieces from A–F to complete the puzzle?

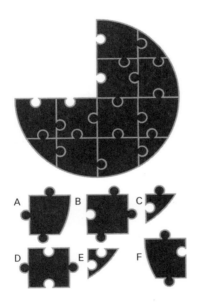

THINKING TIP
Turn to music to improve your thinking. Research has shown that taking music lessons led to an IQ boost in children, and a course of singing lessons resulted in measurable right-brain development in an adult volunteer.

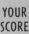
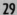

Every Which Way at the Compass

Food at the Compass Dining Rooms is served on square plates with directional arrows, as shown. As part of his induction, new waiter Joseph has to determine which of the four plates A–D below should be chosen to complete the sequence. Can you help him? (Hint: You need to follow each arrow on its course through the plates …)

A B C D

THINKING TIP
If you have to commit a longish number—such as a friend's cellphone number—to memory, try "chunking": Break up the numbers into "chunks" of 2–4 digits (07505184687, say, could be 07 505 184 687).

First Up

Mikhail uses observational challenges like this to determine which quiz team is first up to face questions in the regular college quiz night challenges. The task is to identify the shape that appears in the design only once. Can you do it? He gives the quiz team members 45 seconds.

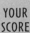
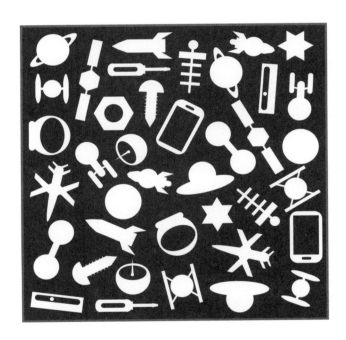

THINKING TIP

Managing your emotions is a key part of good thinking— and smart puzzling. When the going seems tough, don't let frustration or anger cloud your judgment.

Orbital

It's 2095. Aboard the space station *Prospero*, astronauts Miron and Todd have to complete number puzzles on handheld devices to unlock the refrigerated cabinet containing the evening's supplies—the puzzles are to test and maintain clarity of mind. Can you help Miron get his evening meal? The challenge is to link numbers together into groups of 1, 2, or 3 so that the sum of numbers in each group matches one of the totals provided. Some numbers do not belong to a group and must be blanked out. Groups may not touch each other and neither may blanked-out numbers.

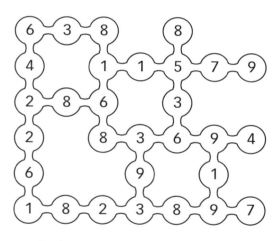

1 . 2 . 3 . 5 . 9 . 13 . 15 . 16 . 19

THINKING TIP
If you're trying the chunking tip on page 30, look for meaningful numbers—in the phone number 01781 215880 you might see the date of the Battle of Yorktown (1781), say, or the sailing of the Spanish Armada against Elizabethan England (1588).

I Am the Gridman

Serial criminal "The Gridman" taunts the police by leaving grid puzzles as his calling card at the scene of the crime. This is one found by Detective Saldano at an art gallery robbery. To solve it you have to shade in cells (the "sea") so that every number is part of a continuous unshaded area (an "island") containing the stated number of cells. There is one number per unshaded island, and islands cannot touch horizontally or vertically (only diagonally); shaded cells cannot form any solid 2x2 (or larger) areas; crucially, all shaded cells must form one continuous area (touching at the corners of cells counts).

			8				
	2			3			
		4				3	
							3
4							
	4				1		
		3				9	
			2				

THINKING TIP
You may be able to improve your ability to visualize in two and three dimensions if you rehearse familiar journeys— say from your office to your car or public transport—in your mind's eye.

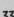

Fool for Figures

Actor Ellis Burroughs specializes in playing the Fool in productions of Shakespeare plays. His acting draws rave reviews but his finances are a mess, so he has taken up doing number puzzles to boost his typically left-brain numerical abilities. Can you help him complete the grid? These are the rules: You have to place the digits 1–9 in the grid so that it's possible to jump from one digit to the next, in order, using the steps provided in the diamonds on the right (for example, the 2,2 in the bottom-right diamond indicates two steps right and two steps down). Each step must be used once, and some refer to numbers already placed. Both parts of a step must be used but can be taken in any order. No part of a step can travel over a black square.

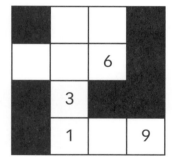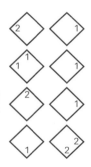

THINKING TIP
Sometimes in everyday mental arithmetic an approximate total is all you need. When a sum seems too hard to do in your head, don't forget you can round up or down; 79 x 41 looks daunting, but 80 x 40 is much easier.

Tango Test

Dance teacher Alejandro surprises students at his evening class by dividing them into pairs and setting them to work on simple puzzles. "It's partly to break the ice," he says, "but also to make people concentrate. In a dance like the tango, you need to be alert and responsive." Here's one of his puzzles. There is a pattern behind the placement of the shaded squares in the grid; can you identify the pattern, and work out what goes in the four squares at A, B, C, and D?

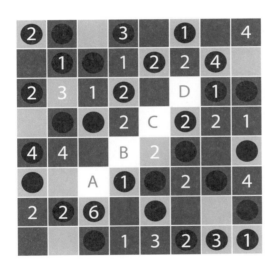

THINKING TIP
Aim for full focus. There are many benefits in giving your whole attention to what you're doing—even to a chore. You'll likely do the task better and enjoy it more.

YOUR
SCORE

Mayan Raid

Games designer Roberto devised this volume puzzle for his video game "Mayana" about Mesoamerican life. A Mayan chieftain discovers that his towering rectangular monument has been attacked and broken down by raiders. The vast brick structure was originally a pile five blocks high, four blocks wide, and five blocks deep and measured 30ft high, 96ft wide, and 50ft deep. Assuming any blocks that can't be seen from this angle are present, can you work out how many bricks remain and their total volume?

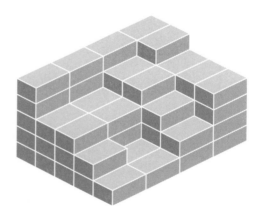

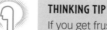

THINKING TIP
If you get frustrated with a puzzle or a problem at work or at home, your annoyance with yourself clouds your thinking and makes it less likely that you'll make progress. It pays to take a break from the job in hand.

Pair Up

An online dating service, Pair Up, loads this number-pairing grid puzzle on its website. Can you solve it? Working from one square to another, horizontally or vertically (never diagonally), you need to draw paths to pair up each set of two matching numbers. No path may be shared, and none may enter a square containing a number or part of another path.

1										2
	3			4	5					
						6	5	4		
				7	8					
				9						10
				6						
						8				
			7		9	1				
								2		
10										3

THINKING TIP
Always maintain a fresh, engaged attitude if you can.
Research has found that people in an upbeat mood are
20 percent more likely to solve a problem requiring insight.

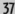

It Fits

In the storeroom at the Food Bank, volunteers David and Marvin invent this number/letter version of a sudoku on a quiet afternoon. The puzzle is played on a 5x5 grid. Each of the twenty-five letter-and-number combinations (from A1 through to E5) appears once in the grid. Each letter and each number must appear once in each row and column. One letter/number combination and some of the letters and numbers are provided.

1		A	C	
	2			3
	B4			
		D		
E		4		

THINKING TIP
Try casting fresh light on a problem by framing it in different terms or viewing it from an opposite perspective.

YOUR
SCORE

Fractions

Fractions is a new agency offering mathematics tuition. Designer Freddie Matisse presents his proposed logos for the agency in the form of a puzzle: A has become B by means of a simple transformation; perform the same transformation on pentagon C and what do you get—D, E, F, or G?

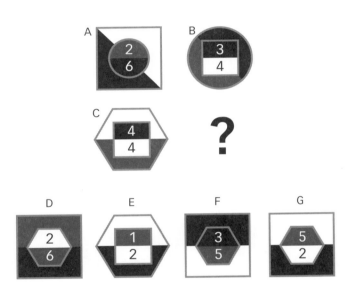

THINKING TIP
Don't always dismiss your gut feeling. Unconscious Thought Theory suggests that when it comes to complex decisions with many variables, the unconscious mind outperforms conscious decision-making.

Encoded

Sports journalist Ben sent this puzzle home to his athletics-mad son Marty. Each number represents a letter. Spell the surnames of seven Olympic champions, then juggle some of the letters to reveal two Olympic host cities. The clues are:

1 1928 men's 5000 meters
2 1968 men's long jump
3 1984 men's 400-meter hurdles
4 2000 women's cycling road race
5 1976 women's all-around gymnastics
6 2008 men's 200 meters
7 2012 women's heptathlon

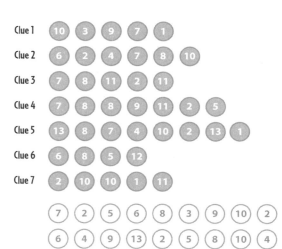

Clue 1   10 3 9 7 1
Clue 2   6 2 4 7 8 10
Clue 3   7 8 11 2 11
Clue 4   7 8 8 9 11 2 5
Clue 5   13 8 7 4 10 2 13 1
Clue 6   6 8 5 12
Clue 7   2 10 10 1 11

7 2 5 6 8 3 9 10 2
6 4 9 13 2 5 8 10 4

THINKING TIP
If you normally take notes as bullet points, try creating a picture or map incorporating the facts you need to record. With visual representations you can use color and position to emphasize sequence and hierarchy.

Router

In his philosophy seminar on determinism and free will, Professor Peters sets this challenge for students Marianne, Tobias, and Ruth. He tells the students, "Draw a path in both grids that passes through every shape exactly once. Paths passing through identical shapes must also be identical. If a shape has been reflected, then its path will also be a mirror image of the corresponding shape in the other grid. The ends of the paths and the starts of the inner routes have been provided."

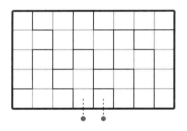

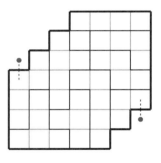

THINKING TIP
If you feel frustration rising, remember it can be part of your thinking process—don't forget that being stuck can be the prelude to a sudden insight or breakthrough (see pages 6–7).

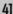

Linkletters

Supermodels Tatiana and Yasmin both got into modeling while studying high-level physics, and one thing that makes them stand out from the crowd is their mutual love of math problems and puzzles. Here's one they work over while waiting for an important runway show in London. The object is to fill the grid with the letters A–F; each row, column, and set of linked circles should contain six different letters.

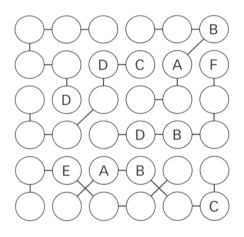

THINKING TIP
Try to be open to information and inspiration from unlikely sources. Be wary of "confirmation bias," a mental habit whereby we tend to discount data with which we don't agree.

Perfect Match

Here's another puzzle that's been uploaded on the Pair Up dating website (see Right Puzzle 10). Can you spot the only two hexagons below that are a perfect match?

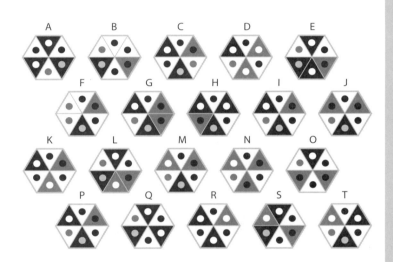

THINKING TIP
Check whether you're thinking in a particular way or making a certain decision in order to fit in. There's a natural tendency to be conformist.

YOUR
SCORE

43

Addshapes

Rivals Zephaniah and Nathaniel are team leaders on a management training day. Can you help Zephaniah's team out-think Nathaniel's on the last challenge of the morning session: Addshapes? These are the rules: The value of each shape is calculated by multiplying the shape's number of sides by the number within it. For example, a triangle containing the number 4 has a value of 12. The task is to find a block of four squares (two squares wide by two squares high) with a total value of 50.

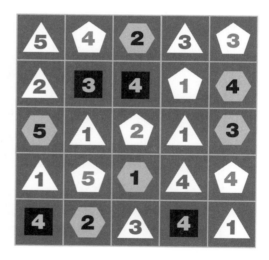

THINKING TIP
Try to limit distractions when working on a problem. Some people swear by completely disconnecting themselves from internet, email, and phone. If that's not possible, try quitting your email program then checking it only once an hour or so.

Memories of Earth

In the year 2175, Gabriel and Michael run a communications center at Lunar Colony Selene XX. The leisure room is filled with games, puzzles, movies, and books, to keep memories of Earth fresh in the lunar colonists' minds. This is an example of one of the simpler puzzles: Can you spot eight differences between the two pictures? Circle them in the picture on the right.

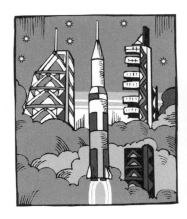

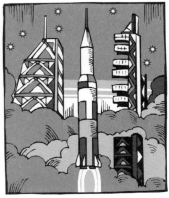

THINKING TIP
Make an effort to combat ingrained habits of thought—for example, about the type of person you are and what you can or can't do, or the jobs/activities you would or would not consider trying.

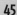

Reverse

Solve the sum 9,800,000 – 2,445,357 then find the answer once within this grid. It occurs in a straight line, running either backward or forward in a horizontal, vertical, or diagonal direction. One catch—as you can see, the numbers are all backward. This puzzle is part of the cover art for author Trudy Kenan's high-finance thriller *Reverse*. Its hero, Henry James, makes $9,800,000 in a deal but then racks up a bill of $2,445,357 celebrating in a champagne bar.

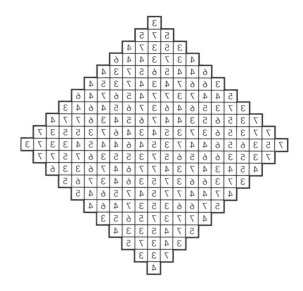

THINKING TIP
One way to build familiarity with numbers and their relations is to revisit your times tables and investigate prime numbers.

Return of the Gridman

Screenwriter Ludovic Rendall has got hold of the true story of serial criminal The Gridman (see Right Puzzle 8) and has dramatized it in a movie, *Follow the Numbers*. Here's one of the puzzles created for the picture: Each number in the grid indicates the exact number of black squares that should surround it; your task is to shade the empty squares until all the numbers are surrounded by the correct number of black squares. In the movie, the fictional detective, Roth, has to count the total black squares, then subtract 3 to extract a key clue.

	3		2	3		4		1
2		4						2
	3			5	6		4	
		3					5	
	4		6		7			1
	5						5	
		4		4		4		
4			2					
	2	2			0		3	

THINKING TIP
You can make it a habit when you're thinking about a challenge to check how well you're concentrating and refocus your attention on the problem in hand.

YOUR
SCORE

Summing Up

Near the beach, Duncan's Café is crowded in season but less busy in winter. In the quiet months, he provides free board games, puzzles, and books for patrons. His Summing Up puzzle is renewed daily and gets quite a name for itself because customers who can solve it in less than 2 minutes win a free homemade ice cream or other dessert if they order a drink. Fancy an ice cream? You have to use the numbers below to complete the six equations shown—three reading across and three reading downward. Every number is used once:

1 2 3 4 5 6 7 8 9

	−		x		=	9
x	■	+	■	x		
	x		−		=	27
x	■	x	■	+		
	x		−		=	43
=		=		=		
126		48		14		

THINKING TIP
Do you like video games? Research suggests that playing them may improve your concentration.

Valley of the Kings

This is a scene from another of Suraj's video games (see Right Puzzle 3). The player takes the role of Edwardian Egyptologist Sir Richard Lymes-Brassington, who has to solve a problem found on a papyrus from the Valley of the Kings in Egypt. Each box should contain one or more symbols from the numbered box to the left of its particular row, plus one or more symbols from the lettered box above its column. However, one square doesn't follow this rule. Which is the odd one out? A bonus is awarded for each symbol you identify as Out of Time for the Egyptian setting.

	A	B	C	D	E	F
	♉ ✪	◇ ◎	⌘ ♈	Ⅱ ♋	↯ ↘	⇐ ⇒
1	↕ ♉ ↔	⇔ ◇	⌘ ⇔ ↕	Ⅱ ↯ ↘	↕ ⇒ ⇐ ↕	
2	☎ ✪ ☏	◎ ☎	♈ ☏ ⌘	☏ Ⅱ	☎ ↯ ↘	☏ ☏ ⇒
3	♉ □ ✪	□ ◇ ◎ ℔	⌘ ♈ ℔	Ⅱ ♋ □	□ ↯	⇐ ℔ ⇒
4	♉ ✧ ✪	◎ ✧ ◇	♈ ✧ ✠	♋ ✧ Ⅱ	✠ ↯ ✧	⇒ ✠ ✧ ⇐
5	↗ ↘	↘ ♉ ↗ ✪	◇ ↘ ◎	↘ ♈ ⌘	♋ ↗ ↘	↗ ⇔ ⇒ ↘	↗ ⇒
6	⇑ ⇓	⇓ ✪	◇ ⇓	⇓ ⌘	Ⅱ ⇓ ⇑ ♋	⇑ ↘ ⇓	⇐ ⇒ ⇑

THINKING TIP
You may be able to prime yourself to discover an insight. Resist getting locked into normal work or problem-solving procedures. Try to be open to unexpected methods and information sources.

YOUR SCORE

Orbital Breakfast

Here's another of the challenges provided on space station *Prospero* to test and maintain the astronauts' mental acuity (see Left Puzzle 8). Miron and Todd have returned to Earth and have been replaced by Arun and Stella. Arun has to solve this puzzle to unlock the compartment containing the morning's supplies. Complete the sudoku grid so that each row and column, and each smaller square of nine cells, contains one each of the nine different shapes. Can you help him get his breakfast?

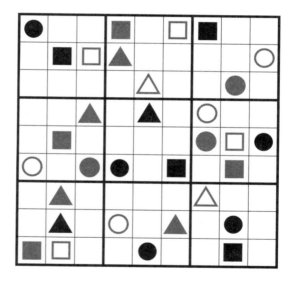

YOUR
SCORE

THINKING TIP

When you get stuck on a puzzle, try shifting your focus to another part. You may be sweating over the gaps in a column when there's an almost-completed row. You can apply this tip—shift focus—more generally when solving problems.

Fare Challenge

Trainee cab driver Wesley Johns knew the format of the City qualification exam was being changed, but he didn't expect—or prepare for—an abstract route puzzle quite like this. Can you help him through this challenge? You have to plot a route along the lines from A to B that avoids all the breaks in the lines. The exam allows you 3 minutes to do it.

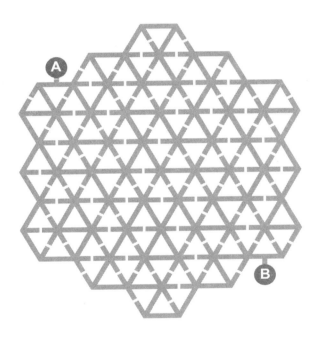

THINKING TIP
Bear in mind the common tendency for people to be "loss averse"—more concerned with avoiding losses than making gains. Is this influencing your thinking or decision-making?

YOUR
SCORE

Zero Smith

Author Edwyn Harrison's publisher creates this puzzle for the interactive ebook edition of his children's classic *Zero Smith*, a story about a young mathematician/private eye. You have to place the numbers 1–9 in each row; numbers may appear multiple times in columns; identical numbers may not appear in neighboring squares—even diagonally. Some diagonal totals are provided around the outside of the grid.

	5	17		20	11			
4		6	8		1	7	5	
	1	5		7	2	4		
21 ◢ 8	2	4			5	3		31 ◣
	3	1		4	9	7		8
23 ◢	4		8		6	5		20 ◣
	3	1	5		9		6	
9 ◢ 4	2		7	3		5	9	17 ◣
	6		1	9	2	7	8	
	4		7	8		1		2

THINKING TIP

When committing numbers to memory, try assigning each of the digits 1–9 a visual image that looks like the number— say a yacht for 4, a cliff for 7. Memory expert Tony Buzan recommends this system for learning and recalling numbers.

YOUR SCORE

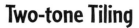

Two-tone Tiling

Mags and Zelda are designing the decor for a new ska and rockin' blues club, and come up with this black and white design for the reception tiling. They know that their friend Wendell, the club owner, enjoys a little puzzling, so they give him this light-hearted challenge: Which of the three sections below does not fit into the main design (tiles may be positioned in any orientation)?

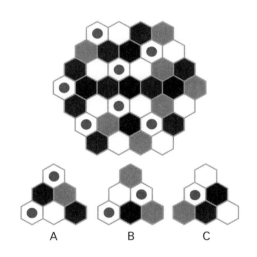

A   B   C

THINKING TIP
People often underestimate their own creativity. To help develop yours, try changing routines or thinking aloud (ask yourself questions), or set yourself deadlines—but don't allow it to stress you out. Above all, be positive!

YOUR
SCORE

LEFT-BRAIN PUZZLE **19** Level 3

Grounded

It's 2099 and the computer module on Dr. Elijah Wilson's flying car is misbehaving—it's making the doctor work through math problems before the ignition will work. This morning the doctor is late for an appointment. Can you help him solve this challenge? Your task is to determine which number should replace the question mark in the outline below.

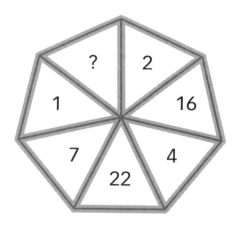

YOUR SCORE

THINKING TIP
You can vary the number-image memory system (see the tip on page 52) by choosing images of things that sound like the names for the numbers in your language.

54

King Bling

Rap star "King Rhymes" is buying a solid-gold crown to wear during his stage show. "What's today's date?" he asks absently, as he prepares to sign a note on his account at the jewelry store. His PA's precocious daughter, Princess, loves teasing Rhymes and replies, "Well ... I was born in the year 2000. The day before yesterday I was nine years old, and next year I'll be 12." What's the date?

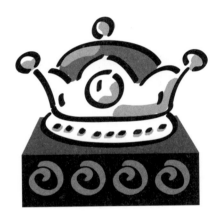

THINKING TIP
Make sure you're focusing on the issue or problem in hand. It's surprisingly common for people to try to solve a related problem that is not really relevant.

YOUR
SCORE

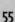

LEFT-BRAIN PUZZLE **20** Level 5

Combiner

Here's another number puzzle from the dressing room of Shakespearean actor Ellis Burroughs (see Left Puzzle 9). Can you solve it? Your task is to place the numbers 1–9 once in each row, column, and 3x3 bold-outlined box. Numbers in circled cells must be equal to the sum of the numbers along the path of their attached arrows.

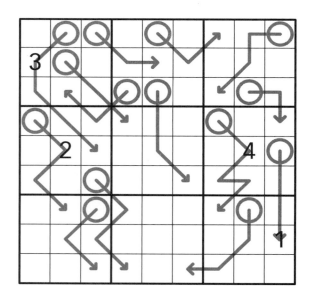

YOUR SCORE

THINKING TIP
One way to gain new perspective is to think of objects in a non-functional way—this can help you see new uses for things or potential new combinations of elements.

56

Cat and Mouse

Super-intelligent, but a little nervous, physics student Samuel likes to have all the bottles neatly and logically arranged when he is working at the Cat and Mouse bar. There are three different designs on the lids of a new sparkling water named "Symbolic," as shown: a triangle, a square, and a star. He's almost finished the display when he's called away to mix a cocktail. Which bottle should we put in to complete his design?

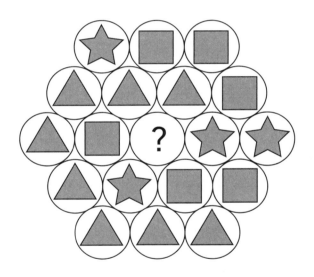

THINKING TIP
Sometimes it pays to limit your choices when making a decision. Psychologists report that people can feel paralyzed by too many options and so fail to decide or make a hurried, random choice not really informed by the available data.

LEFT-BRAIN PUZZLE **21**   Level 4

Four Step

Folk group Waggle Dance use this router puzzle on the cover of their CD single "Ah One, Ah Two, Ah One, Two, Three, Four." Plot a path through the grid that starts in the top-left corner and finishes in the bottom-right. Numbers must link together in the order 1—2—3—4—1—2—3—4 and so on. The path may cross over itself but must visit every number in the grid only once.

1	4	1	2	2	3	4	1
2	3	2	3	1	4	3	2
3	1	4	4	2	3	2	3
1	4	2	3	1	1	4	4
4	2	1	1	3	2	1	1
1	3	4	2	4	3	4	2
3	2	3	1	4	1	2	3
4	1	2	2	3	4	3	4

YOUR
SCORE

THINKING TIP
Psychologists report that we think things more likely to be true if they are easy to process mentally: Sometimes a statement convinces us simply because it's easy. Try restating things in a different way to see if that changes your response.

Quarters

Designer Freddie Matisse (see Right Puzzle 11) presents this divider puzzle when commissioned to create a placemat for the Army Museum restaurant, Quarters. The task for diners is to consider how to divide the grid into four equally sized, equally shaped areas, each of which contains just one each of the four different shapes.

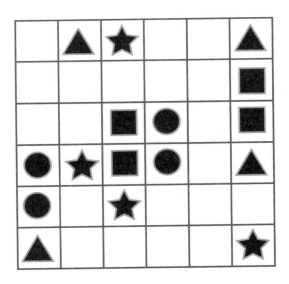

THINKING TIP
In some contexts, deciding you will choose an option that is "good enough" rather than "the best" can simplify decision-making and lead to a good outcome.

YOUR SCORE

Adders

This is one of the harder puzzles provided by dance teacher Alejandro for his students (see Right Puzzle 9). Can you solve it? As in a standard sudoku puzzle, the digits 1–9 are used, and those contained within any set of squares outlined by dots total the number in the lower left-hand corner of the dotted section.

14						14		
			9	10	10			
18			13					
		15	23			23		
	16				14		11	
22			22					
	15				22		14	
			13	25	12			
14	15		18		13	10		

THINKING TIP
Beware "decision fatigue." When we've been thinking hard for a while, we become less likely to make good decisions. Plan to have breaks—or put off finally making a big decision to a time when you know you will be fresh.

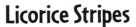

Licorice Stripes

Bagging up licorice candy for the school fair, teacher Mrs. Trainer came up with this idea for a puzzle to run on the stall. There's a prize for all who can solve it: a small bag of candy. The flatplan can be folded to make a cube. Which of the four candies below is the only one it could make?

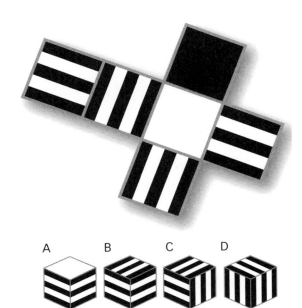

A   B   C   D

THINKING TIP
Don't rush when you're committing something to memory. Focus your full attention when you're inputting facts, to maximize your chance of recalling them later.

YOUR
SCORE

Quiet Night at the Cat and Mouse

At the Cat and Mouse bar, physics student Samuel (see Right Puzzle 20) has made friends with new employee Howie, a math major. On a quiet night, Howie creates this number-symbol puzzle using a handful of beer-bottle tops. Samuel solves it in 2 minutes —can you match his time? Each of the six shapes represents a different number 1–6. Solving the sums left to right and top to bottom, can you work out which shape represents which number? No fractions or negative numbers are involved.

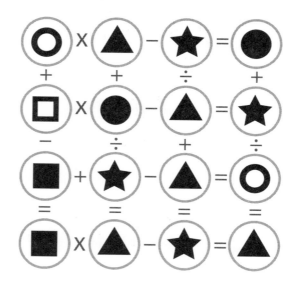

THINKING TIP
Try to put distance between yourself and the matter at hand before making a final decision—this can be distance of time (take a break) or space (go somewhere else). Sometimes this new perspective will throw new light on the issues involved.

Gridman Hits the Precinct

Serial criminal the Gridman (see Right Puzzles 8 and 15) is taunting the cops again—he arranged for the police cars to be reparked in the precinct yard. He's muddled the keys up and sent them back with the following clues: The numbers on the two left-hand cars total the same as the other three. The two odd-numbered cars are adjacent, and every one has moved. Can you help Detective Saldano work out the new arrangement of cars?

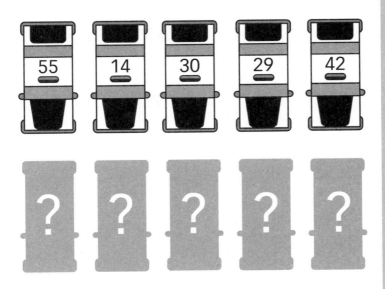

THINKING TIP
Before making a decision, consider whether you're acting for a subjective or an objective reason; imagine yourself in the third person or as a third party looking at a decision.

YOUR
SCORE

Cruise Dice

This is another of movie technician Virgil's dice grids (see Left Puzzle 1). The casino heist movie was a success and a new one was commissioned with the same characters and a similar plot, this time set aboard a cruise liner. Can you solve it? As before, your task is to complete the grid so that dice numbering 1–6 appear in all the rows and all the columns.

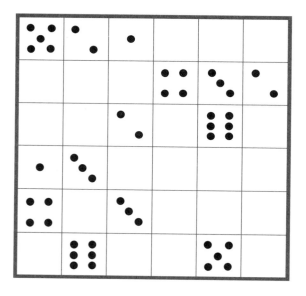

YOUR
SCORE

THINKING TIP
A common element in bad decision-making is that we tend to give too much weight to threats or difficulties that are easy to visualize. Try performing a check—ask yourself, "How likely is that possible bad outcome, really?"

Pot the Black

Rajdeep creates this puzzle for the pool-mad boys at the youth club he manages. Can you hit the black? To succeed, you have to make your way from the cue ball at the top to the black ball, creating a working sum as you go. No negative numbers or fractions are permitted at any point and there is no moving backward.

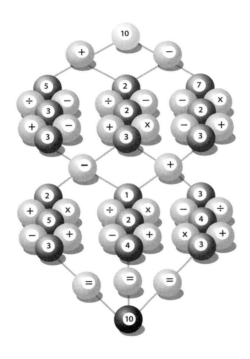

THINKING TIP
One aspect of our preference for things that are easy to process (see the tip on page 58) is our liking for the familiar. In decision-making, try therefore to be open to the unfamiliar.

YOUR
SCORE

Arrow Down

Gentleman aviator Sir Hugo Bonneville crashed his biplane, *The Arrow*, right in the middle of the desert. Sheltering beneath a palm tree, he devised this arrow puzzle. Just like in a traditional sudoku, each row, column, and box of nine smaller squares contains the digits 1–9, but here arrowed lines point toward a smaller number and away from a greater number. Note that 1s can be placed only in squares where all the arrowed lines are pointing inward and 9s can be placed only in squares where all the arrowed lines are pointing outward.

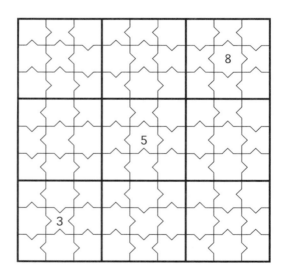

THINKING TIP
Aim for balance—can you identify ways to fulfill parts of yourself that do not find expression in your job or your day-to-day life?

5/4

Here's another of the puzzles enjoyed by supermodels Tatiana and Yasmin (see Left Puzzle 13). As they're waiting to perform in a show at chic club 5/4, Tatiana hands it to her friend and asks, "Can you divide the grid into four equally sized, equally shaped areas, each of which contains just one of each of the five different letters?"

A	B	C	D	E	C
	A				
D		E			
B	C	E		B	
	A	B	C	A	E
		D		D	

THINKING TIP
Try to be adventurous without being rash in your decision-making. Aim for a balance between being open to new opportunities and information and, at the same time, using and developing your discernment to judge between options.

YOUR SCORE

THINKING CHALLENGE 2

Try this second thinking challenge to reassess your left-brain/right-brain thinking, and judge how well you have succeeded in balancing your mental performance in working through this book. We return to the florist's store Joy Blooms (see pages 12–14), where you have been working for a month. Your boss (and family friend) Joy has been delighted with your input, and you're finding the job stimulating— there's outlet for your creativity and you've even received compliments on your eye for color! And your apartment has never been so fragrant or looked so colorful, because Joy encourages her staff to take older blooms home rather than let them go to waste. You haven't missed your previous job at Rainbow Productions, although you did feel one or two twinges of regret when you heard funny tales about the filming of its sitcom in a florist's store …

Flowers, Bills—and Guns!

The last day of the month is pay day at Joy Blooms and the store has unusually large amounts of cash on site. Joy has hired a former broadcasting colleague of yours, Johnnie Roth, to work as a security guard. (For some reason he tells you to give his name as John Book, which puzzles you.)

The day starts with a relatively straightforward problem over bills, but ends with a hold-up!

First, Joy needs you to sort out a billing query—at speed! She's offered a promotion to long-term clients, under which one week's spend in the past month is complimentary. Now Dame Helen Somerville's people are on the line complaining that they've been charged in full for the month. It's the cheapest weekly spend that is complimentary—you don't have a calculator to hand, but can you identify the least expensive week for Joy before Dame Helen herself rings in 5 minutes?

Notes

- Week 1: $49, $93, $125, $439, $212, $73, $39
- Week 2: $512, $34, $90, $399
- Week 3: $125, $215, $512, $95, $33, $21
- Week 4: $111, $97, $54, $45, $45, $73, $65, $55, $310, $32, $43, $55, $75, $56

Toward the end of the day the strangest series of events unfolds, leading to an alarming conclusion … First, after a period of bustle on the sidewalk outside, you notice an unusual quiet. You hear something that sounds like "Packed in!" or perhaps "Action." You wonder if there is a demonstration gathering. Then someone comes in dressed in a clown outfit, and wearing a scarf in all the colors of the rainbow. He asks for some red roses. You serve him:

"Forty-five dollars, please," you say.
"Got any orange tulips?"
"You're in luck," you reply. "That's another sixty-five dollars."
He asks for some sunflowers.
"With pleasure," you say. "That's another seventy-two dollars."

Notes

"Something green?" he asks.

"You could try *Alchemilla*," you suggest. "Lady's mantle. It's ten dollars."

He doesn't seem to respond, indicating with a wave that he can't hear very well. You show him the flowers and he gives a thumbs-up.

Now he says, "I'd like some bluebells or cornflowers."

"With pleasure," you say. "That's fifteen dollars."

Now he looks around the shop. His eyes seize on a flower and he points at it.

"*Baptisia australis*?" You say. "Of course. 'Blue wild indigo.' They're fifty-five dollars."

A note of caution sounds now in your mind. The costs are mounting, and he is so eccentric in appearance. Will he be able to pay? He doesn't look wealthy. He points again.

"Violets?" You say.

He nods again.

"This is an unusual order," you say. "That's another thirty dollars." He is silent, then winks.

Notes

"The total?" You give it to him. (What is it?)

He reaches into his pocket, you assume for a credit card. But he pulls out a gun and points it at you. At this point, like the cavalry riding to the rescue in an old movie, "John Book" walks in. But he doesn't help. Instead, he looks across and smiles.

"Johnnie!" you shout. "The gun?" You almost scream. It is pointing at your chest.

"Morning!" Johnnie calls. But instead of helping, he pulls out a gun himself.

Then the man in the clown outfit pulls the trigger. Out comes a little flag bearing the word "BANG!" Johnnie and the clown laugh. You hear a voice say, "Keep rolling."

You see two cameramen outside the store filming. Then both the clown and Johnnie turn and run out, being filmed all the time. You look around in amazement, think of your life over the past year … and the strangeness of what has happened, and you feel that a moment of insight is about to break in your mind: You will understand what is happening. What is going on?

Notes

THE ANSWERS

The answer section is essential for checking and scoring your responses and plotting your way through the left-brain/right-brain question strands. You may come to your answers after working through all the possible left-brain solutions or following a moment of right-brain insight. Remember after you check your answer to score yourself according to whether you were correct and how easy you found the process (0 for very difficult and incorrect, to 5 for very easy and correct). As mentioned on page 9, if you score 0, 1, or 2, indicating some degree of difficulty, go on to a puzzle of the same kind—for example, from Left 1 to Left 2; if you score 3, 4, or 5, indicating ease and a certain amount of mastery, go on to a puzzle of the opposite kind—for example, from Left 1 to Right 1.

LEFT PUZZLE 1 Casino Dice

The completed grid should look as shown right. If you got this right and found it fairly straightforward to complete, you are strong in typically left-brain activities such as arithmetic and language processing. As explained on pages 9 and 75, if you got it right, award yourself a mark of 3, 4, or 5, depending on how easy you found it (with 5 for very easy), then proceed to Right Puzzle 1. If you couldn't complete the puzzle, score 0, 1, or 2 (award yourself 0 if you found it very difficult); this means you need more practice in left-brain thinking—proceed to Left Puzzle 2.

LEFT PUZZLE 2 Firenze

The completed grid is shown right. The number Paolo needs is 10.

2	16	24	3	17	62
12	15	11	4	19	61
21	5	10	20	6	62
7	22	14	13	18	74
8	9	23	25	1	66
50	67	82	65	61	

LEFT PUZZLE 3 Sir Hector's Code

The missing letter is P (right). The sum total of the values of the letters in the top-left and top-right squares equals that of the central square, as does the sum total of the values of the letters in the bottom-left and bottom-right squares. Thus the missing value is 16 (and P is the 16th letter of the alphabet).

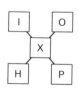

LEFT PUZZLE 4 The Joy of Math

The number grid is shown right.
This puzzle neatly combines mental
arithmetic with number placement.
The club Grace manages is for over-70s
only. Her clients soon find that once
accustomed to the puzzles they take
pleasure in doing them.

8	+	3	−	7	=	4
−		x		+		
1	+	9	−	4	=	6
x			+		−	
6	+	5	x	2	=	22
=		=		=		
42		32		9		

LEFT PUZZLE 5 Whodunit?

The completed loopline is
shown right. Gilbert finds
the puzzles relaxing when
his head is full of plot twists
and considerations of where
to reveal key information in
the narrative.

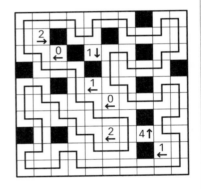

LEFT PUZZLE 6 Davy's Dice

The final die in your trip is the dark gray 4, the second die in the top row.
The directions are as follows: white = up; dark gray = down; black = left;
light gray = right.

LEFT PUZZLE 7 Every Which Way at the Compass

The answer is C, shown right. Each symbol follows a
path over the course of the plates that takes it (one
square at a time) down the first column, then up the
central column, then down the right column. When a
symbol reaches the bottom-right position, it moves to the top-left corner
of the next box. Joseph passes the test and gets the job. At college he
majors in mathematics, so he is well primed in the left-brain skills needed
to pass such challenges. It pays to be prepared.

↗	↙	⇐
⇐	⇧	↓
↘	↖	⇨

LEFT PUZZLE 8   Orbital

The correct grouping of numbers is shown right. The top-left group, for example, totals 13. Todd, a New Yorker, is strong in left-brain processing and always aces the number puzzles, but Miron—from Siberia—is stronger at visual challenges. They're both working at balancing their thinking.

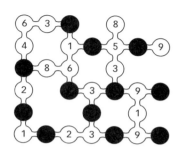

LEFT PUZZLE 9   Fool for Figures

The numbers 1–9 should fit in the grid as seen here.

	4	5	
7	8	6	
	3		
	1	2	9

LEFT PUZZLE 10   Mayan Raid

Each brick measures 6 x 24 x 10ft, making a volume of 1,440ft³; 67 bricks remain; 67 x 1,440ft³ = 96,480ft³. If you found it easy to work out this fairly tricky calculation, then your left-brain thinking is strong.

LEFT PUZZLE 11   It Fits

The completed grid is shown right. David and Marvin's puzzle tests typically left-brain logic and sequencing. There are quite a few math and physics students among the volunteers, all of whom swap puzzles freely.

B1	D3	A2	C5	E4
D4	C2	B5	E1	A3
A5	B4	E3	D2	C1
C3	E5	D1	A4	B2
E2	A1	C4	B3	D5

LEFT PUZZLE 12   Encoded

Marty aced the challenge, even though he was able to fill in only a single clue as a starting point, and sent his dad the following answers: 1 = I; 2 = E; 3 = U; 4 = A; 5 = L; 6 = B; 7 = M; 8 = O; 9 = R; 10 = N; 11 = S; 12 = T; 13 = C. The champions are: 1. Paavo NURMI; 2. Bob BEAMON; 3. Ed MOSES; 4. Leontien Zijlaard-van MOORSEL; 5. Nadia COMANECI; 6. Usain BOLT; 7. Jessica ENNIS. The two Olympic cities are: MELBOURNE and BARCELONA. How did you do? A good performance means you're strong in left-brain verbal/numerical dexterity.

LEFT PUZZLE 13   Linkletters

Tatiana and Yasmin's completed grid is shown right. The Religious Society of Friends' (or Quakers) book *Advices & Queries* includes this useful advice that links to the idea of confirmation bias (see tip): "Listen patiently and seek the truth which other people's opinions may contain for you …
Do not allow the strength of your convictions to betray you into making statements or allegations that are unfair or untrue. Think it possible that you may be mistaken."

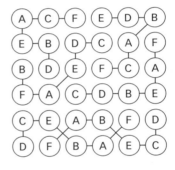

LEFT PUZZLE 14   Addshapes

As shown (right), the section is toward the top right of the grid, containing a 1-pentagon (5), a 4-hexagon (4 x 6 = 24), a 1-triangle (3), and a 3-hexagon (3 x 6 = 18); 5 + 24 + 3 + 18 = 50. How did you find this puzzle? It tests your powers of observation in tandem with quick mental arithmetic.

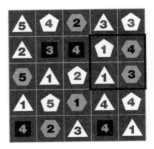

LEFT PUZZLE 15 Reverse

9,800,000 − 2,445,357 = 7,354,643. You can find this number in the grid as shown. Author, mathematician, and memory expert Daniel Tammet has an intense familiarity with numbers, in part because as a child with Asperger's syndrome (a form of autism) and few friends, he thought about them a great deal. He also has synesthesia, and experiences digits as having colors and even textures. For him, numbers are connected in a web in the same way that words are in a language. He argues that we can all have a more familiar and engaged relationship with numbers by changing our attitude to mathematics, and thinking about them more.

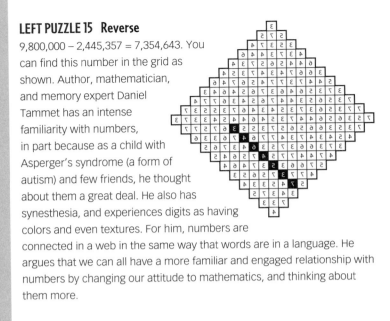

LEFT PUZZLE 16 Summing Up

The completed grid is shown right. Did you manage it in less than 2 minutes?

3	−	2	×	9	=	9
×		+		×		
7	×	4	−	1	=	27
×		×		+		
6	×	8	−	5	=	43
=		=		=		
126		48		14		

LEFT PUZZLE 17 Orbital Breakfast

The completed grid is shown right. Arun complains to the onboard computer Miranda that this provides quite a test of his eye for detail and sequential processing so soon after waking, but Miranda counters that the astronauts are expected to be in a state of readiness on the space station.

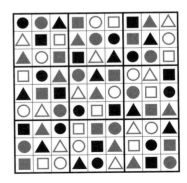

LEFT PUZZLE 18
Zero Smith

The completed grid is shown right. The idea of right- and left-brain thinking is prominent in Harrison's book: Zero tries to engage his whole brain on problems— although he is naturally gifted in left-brain numerical and logical

		5	17		20	11		
4	2	6	8	3	1	7	5	9
3	1	5	9	7	2	4	8	6
8	2	4	6	1	5	3	9	7
5	3	1	2	4	9	7	6	8
1	4	9	8	7	6	5	2	3
8	3	1	5	2	9	7	4	6
4	2	8	7	3	6	5	9	1
5	3	6	4	1	9	2	7	8
6	4	5	7	8	3	1	9	2

(21, 23, 9 on the left; 31, 20, 17 on the right)

thinking, he makes a deliberate effort to bring right-brain insights to bear on the cases he has to solve.

LEFT PUZZLE 19 Grounded

The answer is 11, as shown. Starting at 1 and moving clockwise, jump over one segment at a time and add 1, then 2, then 3, then 4, then 5, then 6. This is a test of typically left-brain numerical logic, but some lateral thinking is involved, as your starting point is not the most obvious.

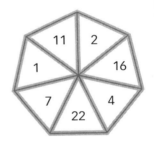

LEFT PUZZLE 20 Combiner

The completed grid is as shown right. The Combiner arrows add a tricky element to an already difficult number-placement puzzle, testing left-brain arithmetic and logic. Before playing Nick Bottom in *A Midsummer Night's Dream*, Ellis receives a call from his accountant, Graeme Hockney, to congratulate him on getting his financial papers in much better order this year.

2	8	5	7	6	3	4	1	9
3	7	9	4	1	2	8	5	6
1	4	6	8	9	5	3	7	2
8	3	4	1	2	7	9	6	5
6	2	1	5	3	9	7	4	8
5	9	7	6	8	4	1	2	3
7	1	8	3	5	6	2	9	4
4	5	2	9	7	8	6	3	1
9	6	3	2	4	1	5	8	7

LEFT PUZZLE 21 Four Step

The route is shown right. After the success of their single, Waggle Dance print both question and answer versions on the cover of their album, "On the Somerset Levels." Lead singer Tick is very keen on left-brain/right-brain thinking and is eager to include puzzles in the band's promo materials.

LEFT PUZZLE 22 Adders

The completed grid is shown right. Like Left Puzzles 1 and 17, this tests and develops typically left-brain positional logic. Doing puzzles of this kind should improve your working memory and powers of concentration.

LEFT PUZZLE 23
Quiet Night at the Cat and Mouse

The key is as follows: solid circle (top right) = 6; hollow circle (top left) = 5; star = 4; solid square (bottom left) = 3; triangle = 2; hollow square (left column, 2nd down) = 1. The completed sums should be as shown right. This is a simple test of mathematical logic.

$$5 \times 2 - 4 = 6$$
$$1 \times 6 - 2 = 4$$
$$3 + 4 - 2 = 5$$
$$3 \times 2 - 4 = 2$$

LEFT PUZZLE 24   Cruise Dice

Virgil's completed grid is shown right. If you found this very difficult last time, how did this puzzle compare? You should find, as you work through the book, that the type of thinking you initially found hardest becomes more manageable.

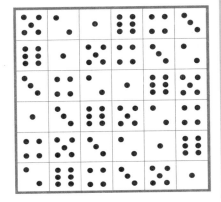

LEFT PUZZLE 25
Arrow Down

The completed grid looks as shown right. With only three digits provided, this is a pretty tough number-placement challenge, providing a stern test of left-brain digital skills. As you've no doubt found on this and similar puzzles, it is sometimes useful to pencil in alternatives for each square. Sir Hugo later credited his

5	1	8	2	3	6	7	4	9
7	2	6	9	4	5	1	8	3
9	4	3	1	8	7	2	5	6
6	7	4	3	2	9	5	1	8
3	8	9	4	5	1	6	7	2
1	5	2	6	7	8	3	9	4
4	6	1	5	9	2	8	3	7
8	3	5	7	6	4	9	2	1
2	9	7	8	1	3	4	6	5

decision to devise some puzzles for his nephew Myles with saving his sanity in the desert; in time he was rescued by a passing camel-herder and helped as far as the coast, from where he sent this and other puzzles to Myles. The adventurer had to leave his beloved *Arrow* behind.

RIGHT PUZZLE 1
Taking It Easy

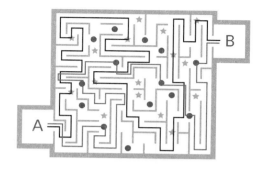

The correct route from A to B and back again is shown right. The puzzle tests and develops typically right-brain spatial perception, the ability to see how things fit together. (See the answer to Right Puzzle 14 for more on this.) How did you find this puzzle? As explained on pages 9 and 75, if you managed to complete it, award yourself a mark of 3, 4, or 5 depending on how easy you found it (with 5 for very easy), then proceed to Left Puzzle 1. If you didn't manage it, score 0, 1, or 2 depending on how much it baffled you (with 0 for really baffled); this means you need more practice in right-brain thinking—proceed to Right Puzzle 2.

RIGHT PUZZLE 2   Colors Fade

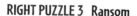

The missing section is C. Each row and column contains one design with three black and three light gray pieces, one with three black and three dark gray pieces, and one with three light gray and three dark gray pieces. Each row and column also has one design that is turned through 90 degrees. The missing design should have three black and three light gray pieces and be turned through 90 degrees.

RIGHT PUZZLE 3   Ransom

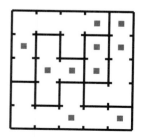

The completed grid is shown right. This level of Suraj's video game provides a good work-out for typically right-brain visual and spatial perception. Finishing this level, you're granted access to another on which the player has to assemble a 3D jigsaw.

RIGHT PUZZLE 4
Path of Attraction

The first flower is the middle bloom in the right column. The entire sequence of flowers visited by the butterfly is shown right. Heather, strong in right-brain visualization, arrived at the answer by working backward. She began taking an interest in mathematics in an attempt to balance her thinking.

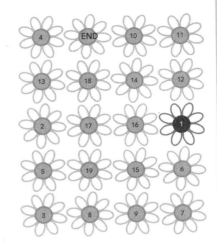

RIGHT PUZZLE 5 A Symbol Problem

The missing piece is B, as shown. Where shapes touch an adjacent square at a certain point, the shape in that adjacent square must also touch there. If you found it easy to work out which part fits within the whole in the grid, then your right-brain thinking is strong.

RIGHT PUZZLE 6 Jigsaw Aria

A, B, E, and F, as shown (right). It's not such a crisis as it might seem, because Roddy and Benedict both have plenty of visual and spatial intelligence, a typically right-brain strength, and they are able to fit the puzzle together before the end of the aria. Now they just need to dream up a suitably creative way to get their own back on Jonathan.

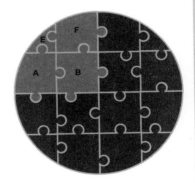

RIGHT PUZZLE 7   First Up

The singleton piece is shown right. Did you manage it within 45 seconds?

RIGHT PUZZLE 8   I Am the Gridman

Detective Saldano's completed grid, satisfying all of the Gridman's conditions, is shown to the right. Can you find any possible variations that also work?

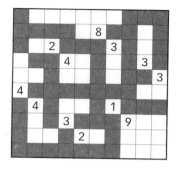

RIGHT PUZZLE 9   Tango Test

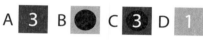

The missing squares A–D are shown right. Each row and column in the grid should contain three light gray and five dark gray squares, four black circles, and numbers that total ten. The puzzle engages you in right-brain thinking about the setting for individual elements, and how items in a pattern fit together.

RIGHT PUZZLE 10   Pair Up

The numbers can be paired as shown here—you may find other possible routes. The puzzle tests typically right-brain visual acuity. Completing the grid on the website wins you a ticket to a complimentary speed-dating evening at Pair Up's headquarters.

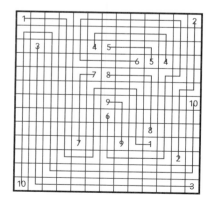

RIGHT PUZZLE 11 Fractions

G. The inside and outside shapes and colors have switched and the color position is reversed. The top number has increased by 1 and the bottom number has decreased by 2. Unconscious Thought Theory (see the tip) was developed by Ap Dijksterhuis and Loran Nordgren in 2006. The theory indicates that it can be unproductive to overthink a problem.

RIGHT PUZZLE 12 Router

The two correct paths are shown below. Professor Peters' puzzle tests awareness of setting and how things connect. In the seminar the students discuss evidence from neuroscience suggesting that your brain prepares you for an action before you make a conscious decision to perform the action—so how can you be said to be acting freely?

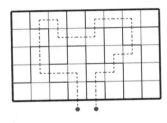
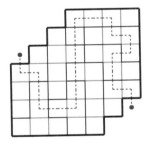

RIGHT PUZZLE 13 Perfect Match

Only I and P are identical. Pair Up loads the puzzle on its website as part of a promotion: Solve the puzzle to win tickets for the website's Manhattanite Walk in Central Park. With regard to conformity (see tip), sometimes you may also benefit from checking that you're not thinking or deciding in a particular way in order *not* to fit in. Clear-minded thinking involves being sure you're deciding/dealing with the problem in hand and not being influenced by all kinds of extraneous matters.

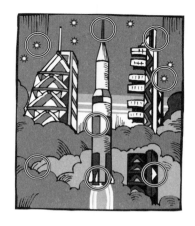

RIGHT PUZZLE 14
Memories of Earth

The eight differences are as shown (right). In your right brain you typically process awareness of how the elements in a picture or scene fit together—the type of thinking tested by "spot the difference" challenges like this. Recognizing a familiar face is a similar right-brain activity. When you recognize a face you assess how facial elements—nose, ears, eyes, and so on—fit together into a known whole. Research at University College London in 2004 identified the right fusiform gyrus as the brain region particularly involved in recognizing a face.

RIGHT PUZZLE 15
Return of the Gridman

The shaded grid is shown right. The total number of shaded squares is 37; 37 − 3 = 34. Detective Roth finds out that the Gridman's next crime is near the Empire State Building on 34th St. in Manhattan. This makes for a great set piece in the movie.

RIGHT PUZZLE 16   Valley of the Kings

The odd one out is E5, as neither of the column E symbols appear. How many Out of Time symbols did you find? Certainly the telephone, and perhaps the question mark. Once he solves the problem, Sir Richard proceeds to a lower level of the tomb, in which he finds a time machine that carries him back to the 21st century.

RIGHT PUZZLE 17
Fare Challenge

The completed route is shown right. After spending several months establishing routes and committing them to memory, Wesley is strong in typically right-brain processing of this type and, although the puzzle surprises him, he has little difficulty in working out the route within the permitted 3 minutes.

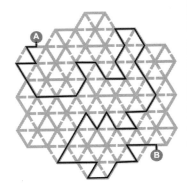

RIGHT PUZZLE 18 Two-tone Tiling

Sections B and C fit as shown; section A is the odd one out. Wendell is good at figures and making a deal; he's less strong in visual thinking, and Zelda tells him the challenge will boost his right-brain performance.

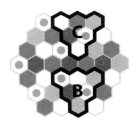

RIGHT PUZZLE 19 King Bling

The date is January 1, 2011. Princess's birthday is on December 31 and yesterday she turned ten. She was nine on December 30, she will be eleven the following December, and twelve the following year. If you didn't get it right first time, look out for other number riddles and get as much practice as you can. Daniel Tammet (see also answer to Left Puzzle 15), an "autistic savant"—one of a group of people with autism who have remarkable abilities—reckons we all potentially have the same abilities. Intriguingly, Australian researcher Allan Snyder conducted experiments that suggest we do all have the astounding powers exhibited by savants, but that, in the majority of people, cognitive thinking overrides and limits these abilities. Snyder's tests interrupt cognitive functioning in volunteers using magnetic pulses—drawing or mathematics skills markedly increased among the test subjects.

RIGHT PUZZLE 20
Cat and Mouse

A square. Then every triangle of six circles, whichever way up, contains one of one shape, two of another, and three of the third.

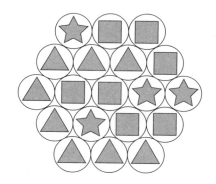

RIGHT PUZZLE 21 Quarters

The grid should be divided into four as shown. The Army Museum is pleased with Freddie's design and it is soon in place in the Quarters restaurant.

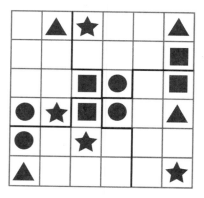

RIGHT PUZZLE 22 Licorice Stripes

The correct answer is B (right). Seeing how the parts fit together in the whole is a key aspect of right-brain processing—see also the answer to Right Puzzle 14.

RIGHT PUZZLE 23 Gridman Hits the Precinct

The new arrangement of cars is shown below. This tests your grasp of spatial logic and simple math.

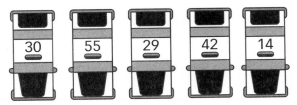

RIGHT PUZZLE 24
Pot the Black

10 + 5 (15) ÷ 3 (5) + 3 (8) − 1 (7) x 2 (14) − 4 = 10. The route from cue ball to black ball is shown right. The boys at Rajdeep's youth club can be resistant to math-related thinking, but he is keen to help them develop numerical confidence, so he often—as here—couches a problem in an appealing everyday setting.

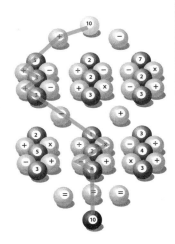

RIGHT PUZZLE 25 5/4

The four sections—each looking a little like a question mark—are shown right. Like a form of jigsaw puzzle, Tatiana's fitment challenge tests and develops typically right-brain consideration of how elements combine in their setting. After the show, Yasmin and Tatiana have a meeting with a journalist from a popular science magazine and agree to start a column, "From the Runway," containing their puzzles and thoughts on recreational math.

A	B	C	D	E	C
	A				
D		E			
B	C	E		B	
	A	B	C	A	E
		D		D	

THINKING CHALLENGE 1 In Bloom

Quite a challenging first day in your job! The way in which you set about memorizing the directions to Dame Helen's hotel will be revealing of your habitual thinking style. A left-brain approach is to memorize the street names—like this: north on Ridgeway, right on Oyster, left on Yale … A right-brainer would focus more on the landmarks—as follows: north from the shop, right at Screen World, left at the cathedral … Which approach did you take?

How would you fare assembling a display unit without instructions? Some people are good at seeing how things fit together and are able to bypass the instructions even when they are available. This is a right-brain skill. Others need to follow each step in the printed instructions to have any chance of producing a workable unit. This is a left-brain approach. If you're in the second group—and stuck without assembly instructions—a creative response (perhaps relying on right-brain intuitive thinking) is to go online and search the product code. You may well be able to download the assembly instructions for printing or perhaps load them on your smartphone and follow them step by step in that way.

For the second delivery, how did you fare in learning the numbers? Did it help you to visualize a hand entering the codes into the keypad? The left brain processes sequences and numerical elements, so if you simply commit the number codes to memory, your typical thinking style is chiefly reliant on your left brain. But when you visualize a hand entering the codes you might notice shapes, identifiable as the Roman numerals L (50), X (10), and M (1,000): 14789 makes the shape of L, 159753 makes an X shape, and 7415369 makes the shape M. If you rely on these shapes rather than the sequence of digits, this suggests you generally depend more on right-brain processing. (You might well, of course, remember the shape made by the number sequence without identifying it as that of a letter or Roman numeral.)

For the final task, would you feel confident about making up bouquets? If you have a natural facility to combine shapes and colors in a pleasing display, this would suggest that you are strong in right-brain processing. If you're more of a left-brainer, you're likely to ask for instructions from Joy or from another coworker, or to look for help in a book or on a website. If you stay in the job, there is no doubt—since practice improves facility and we can all remake our thinking preferences—that you will improve as a flower-arranger as you are asked to make up orders over the following weeks.

For each of the four elements of the challenge:
- If you strongly favor right-brain processing score 3.
- If you mildly favor right-brain processing score 2.
- If you strongly favor left-brain processing score 1.
- If you mildly favor left-brain processing score 0.

Left-Brain/Right-Brain Questionnaire
Questions 1, 2, 4, 7, 9: If you agree, you tend more toward right-brain processing. Score 2 for each question you ticked.

Questions 3, 5, 6, 8, 10: If you ticked these, you tend more toward left-brain processing. Score 1 for each question you ticked.

Combine your score for Thinking Challenge 1 with your score on the questionnaire to get your Starting Score. Our aim is to balance your thinking, so if your score indicates you are strong in right-brain thinking, start with a left-brain puzzle. Conversely, if your score suggests you excel at left-brain tasks, begin with a right-brain puzzle.

- **If you scored 18–27** start with Left Puzzle 1.
- **If you scored 10–17** start with either Left or Right Puzzle 1.
- **If you scored 0–9** start with Right Puzzle 1.

THINKING CHALLENGE 2   Flowers, Bills—and Guns!
The cheapest week is Week 3. These are the totals: Week 1— $1,030; Week 2—$1,035; Week 3—$1,001; Week 4—$1,116. You manage to work out the totals in time to tell Joy before Dame Helen rings. You also manage to keep a running total in your encounter with the clown ($292).

After John and the clown run from the store you feel very angry. As for the supposedly comical hold-up, you experience a sense of impasse. You really cannot make sense of this. You think back to how the clown seemed to be prompting you to consider the order. Looking at the flowers on your desk the word "rainbow" comes to mind, then—looking more closely—you see that the flowers he asked for are in the colors of the rainbow: red/orange/yellow/green/blue/indigo/violet. Of course, this word reminds you of the broadcasting company you and Johnnie used to work for. Weren't they making a show about a florist's store? And there was a cameraman outside. Did you hear the words "Action" and "Keep rolling"? When you go outside you find that a film crew is there, still filming … The scene is an insert to be included in the company's florist's store sitcom. When you tackle Johnnie about it he claims he tried to give you a clue by calling himself John Book—the name, he says, of the cop who goes under a hidden identity among the Amish in Peter Weir's 1985 movie *Witness*.

Ability with numbers, as we have seen elsewhere, is typically left-brain thinking. The capacity to get an overview of the encounter with the clown, to see things from outside your own immediate perspective, on the other hand, is typically right-brain thinking. Which type do you find easier? You have no doubt developed a clear idea of where you are naturally more at ease; in this book you have worked through puzzles and thinking challenges designed to support and improve your mental performance in areas that come less naturally to you—in order to balance your mental life. Logical people can benefit from learning to trust their intuition more, just as people of a creative, instinctive disposition will often be glad to add clarity of thinking and numerical confidence to their mental arsenal.

How Did You Do?

Now that you've worked your way through the book, why not count up how many of each number you scored to get an idea of your overall performance? Here's an idea of what it means:

- Mostly 5s—you're a genius! Your thinking is balanced but it never hurts to get more practice.
- Mostly 4s—pretty impressive. Maybe you found some of the puzzles a bit tricky, but you got there in the end.
- Mostly 3s—well done, you persevered. Even if you struggled with some puzzles, you kept going. You're on the way to balancing your thinking.
- Mostly 2s—good effort. You didn't give up, even if some of the puzzles got the better of you. Keep trying and you'll find you begin to improve.
- Mostly 1s—practice makes perfect. The more you stretch your brain, the more you'll fine-tune your thinking and the greater the benefits.
- Mostly 0s—don't be disheartened. Perhaps most of the puzzles had you stumped, but keep stretching your brain and you will notice a difference.

Further Reading & Resources

Books

"Bertie changes his mind," from *Carry On, Jeeves* by P.G. Wodehouse, Herbert Jenkins 1925

Descartes' Error: Emotion, Reason, and the Human Brain by Antonio Damasio, Vintage 2006

How to Stay Sane by Philippa Perry/ The School of Life, Pan Macmillan 2012

Humanity on a Tightrope: Thoughts on Empathy, Family, and Big Changes for a Viable Future by Paul R. Ehrlich and Robert E. Ornstein, Rowman & Littlefield 2012

Imagine: How Creativity Works by Jonah Lehrer, Canongate 2012

Left Brain Right Brain by Charles Phillips, Connections Books 2010

Right Hand, Left Hand by Chris McManus, Phoenix 2003

Self Comes to Mind: Constructing the Conscious Brain by Antonio Damasio, Vintage 2012

Stairway of Surprise by Michael Lipson, Anthroposophic Press 2002

The New Drawing on the Right Side of the Brain by Betty Edwards, Harper Collins 2001

The Right Mind: Making Sense of the Hemispheres by Robert E. Ornstein, Harcourt 1998

The Tell-Tale Brain by V.S. Ramachandran, Random House India 2010

The Valley of Fear by Sir Arthur Conan Doyle, George H. Doran 1915

Thinking, Fast and Slow by Daniel Kahneman, Penguin 2012

Thinking in Numbers: How Maths Illuminates Our Lives by Daniel Tammet, Hodder & Stoughton 2013

Games

Left Brain Right Brain 2 (Nintendo DS)
Puzzler—Mind Gym (Nintendo 3DS)

Article

"The Eureka Hunt" by Jonah Lehrer, in *The New Yorker*, July 28, 2008

Websites

Meditation guidance: www.easwaran.org

Quaker Faith & Practice (*Advices & Queries*): www.qfp.quakerweb.org.uk/qfp1-02.html

Seed Magazine: www.seedmagazine.com

The School of Life: www.theschooloflife.com

The Author

Charles Phillips is the author of more than 30 books, including *Stay Smart* (2012), the Brain Builder series, and *Business Brain Trainer* (both 2011), as well as eight volumes in the best-selling *How to Think* series (2009–13). Charles has also investigated Indian theories of intelligence and consciousness in *Ancient Civilizations* (2005), probed the brain's dreaming mechanism in *My Dream Journal* (2003), and examined how we perceive and respond to color in his *Colour for Life* (2004).

EDDISON•SADD EDITIONS
Concept Nick Eddison
Managing Editor Tessa Monina
Designer Brazzle Atkins
Production Sarah Rooney

BIBELOT LTD
Editor Ali Moore
Puzzle-checker Sarah Barlow

PUZZLE PROVIDERS
Guy Campbell; Clarity Media;
Laurence May, Vexus Puzzle Design; Puzzle Press